TUBAL LIGATION RECOVERY COOKBOOK

Complete Guide Unlocking The Secrets Of
Nutrition To Rapid Healing After Surgery
Success, Nourishing Meal Plans, Recipes, Tips
For Optimal Health Wellness

DR. ALLAN FREDA

Contents

This cookbook is all about helping them get better by giving them the best diet after surgery.

In the book, there are healing recipes that are meant to help people get better, as well as carefully planned meal plans to make sure they eat well during this important time. In addition, long-term wellness tips from experts are given, which can help you live a healthy life after the recovery process is over. This recipe is very helpful for people who are going through the process of healing after tubal ligation surgery because it focuses on healthy eating and nourishing the body.

Disclaimer

The information in this book is for informational purposes only and should not replace professional medical advice, diagnosis, or treatment. Always consult your physician or a qualified health provider regarding any medical concerns. Do not disregard professional medical advice or delay seeking it based on information in this book.

The author does not endorse or have affiliations with any mentioned entities. References are for informational purposes only.

Consult your healthcare provider before making dietary or lifestyle changes, especially during recovery from surgery, as individual needs vary.

Results may vary, and the information provided is not guaranteed to produce specific outcomes.

By reading this book, you acknowledge and agree to consult your healthcare provider before implementing any information herein.

For further guidance, consult your healthcare provider or reputable medical websites for reliable information on surgery recovery diets.

CHAPTER 1
AN INTRODUCTION TO TUBERCULOSIS RECOVERY

Tubal ligation, which is also known as "getting your tubes tied," is a surgery that many people choose when they want to permanently stop having children. The fallopian tubes are blocked, sealed, or cut during this process so that eggs can't get from the ovaries to the uterus to be fertilized.

Even though tubal ligation is usually thought to be safe and effective, the body still needs time to heal properly afterward.

How to Understand Surgery for Tubal Ligation:

Several methods, such as laparoscopy or mini-laparotomy, can be used to do tubal closure surgery. For laparoscopic tubal ligation, which is the most common way, small cuts are made in the abdomen. A thin, lit tube with a camera (laparoscope) and surgical tools are then put through these cuts. Then, clips, rings, or cauterization are used to stop or close off the fallopian tubes. A mini-laparotomy makes a bigger cut in the belly and is usually only done on people who have had abdominal surgery before or who have certain medical conditions.

 No matter what method is used, tubal ligation is thought to be a pretty small surgery with a low risk of complications.

It is very important to get enough nutrients while recovering from tubal ligation surgery. The body needs certain vitamins, minerals, and nutrients to help repair tissues, lower inflammation and speed up healing generally.

Getting enough food can also help with common problems that come up after surgery, like feeling tired, sick, or unable to go to the toilet. A healthy diet can also help keep hormone levels in check and improve sexual health, which may be especially important for people whose hormones are changing because of surgery.

How this cookbook can help you get better:

The Tubal Ligation Recovery Cookbook is a complete guide to healthy eating after surgery. It is designed to meet the unique nutritional needs of people who are recovering from tubal ligation.

This recipe has a lot of useful information on healthy foods, meal plans, and long-term health tips from experts.

Whether you've just been told and are getting ready for surgery or are already in the recovery process, this cookbook will help you a lot.

This cookbook gives people the tools they need to take care of their health and well-being during this important time, with recipes that are high in nutrients and practical tips on how to deal with symptoms after surgery.

With its focus on healthy foods and meals, the Tubal Ligation Recovery Cookbook gives you all the tools you need to speed up your recovery, feel better, and start living a healthier life after surgery.

CHAPTER 2
GIVING YOUR BODY WHAT IT NEEDS

A good diet is very important for people who have recently had surgery, including those who have had tubal ligation. A healthy, varied diet not only helps the body heal itself, but it also gives you more energy and makes you feel better overall. It is very important to know what nutrients you need to recover because they are very important for healing tissues, keeping your immune system healthy, and your general health.

Important Nutrients for Healing:

After tubal ligation surgery, the body goes through several changes that help it heal and get better.

At this time, it is very important to get enough of the foods your body needs, like vitamins, minerals, and antioxidants.

These nutrients help biochemical processes happen that are important for healing tissues and the immune system. For example, vitamin C helps make collagen, which is an important part of healing wounds, and zinc boosts the immune system and encourages cell repair. Vitamin E is also a strong antioxidant that protects cells from environmental damage and speeds up the healing process. Including a range of nutrient-dense foods in the diet after surgery, like fruits, veggies, whole grains, lean proteins, and healthy fats, will make sure that the body gets enough of these important nutrients.

Adding foods high in protein:

Protein is very important for healing after surgery because it gives tissues and muscles the building blocks they need to grow back. Eating a lot of protein-rich foods can help you heal faster and keep your muscles from losing mass. Lean meats, chicken, fish, eggs, dairy products, legumes, nuts, and seeds are all good sources of high-quality protein.

It is important for tissue repair and immune system function that you eat these foods at meals and as snacks throughout the day. They provide a steady supply of amino acids, which are the building blocks of protein. Protein-rich foods also help you feel full and keep your blood sugar levels steady, which is good for your general health and energy while you're recovering.

Healthy Fats for the Best Healing:

Fats have been criticized in the past, but they are very important for health, especially after surgery when the body is still healing. Healthy fats give you a lot of energy and carry fat-soluble vitamins like A, D, E, and K to your cells, where they're needed for immune system health and tissue repair.

Adding healthy fats to your diet, like those found in avocados, olive oil, nuts, seeds, and fatty fish, helps you heal better and stay healthy over time. Fatty fish like salmon and trout contain omega-3 fatty acids, which are anti-inflammatory and can help reduce pain and swelling after surgery. Adding different kinds of healthy fats to meals also makes them taste better and make you feel fuller, which makes it easier to stick to a healthy diet while you're recovering.

Fibre and staying hydrated are important parts of nutrition after surgery that are often forgotten, but they are also very important for healing and general health. Fibre helps keep your digestive system healthy and helps you have normal bowel movements, which can be messed up by surgery and some painkillers.

Fiber-rich foods like fruits, veggies, whole grains, and legumes can help keep you from getting constipated and make your digestive system feel better while you're healing. Additionally, staying hydrated is important for wound healing because it helps blood flow and delivers nutrients to damaged tissues. Along with eating foods that are high in water, like fruits and veggies, drinking a lot of water throughout the day helps the body stay properly hydrated and heal itself.

Finally, it is very important to keep your body healthy after tubal ligation surgery by eating a varied diet full of protein, healthy fats, fiber, and water. People can support their bodies' natural healing processes and improve their long-term health by focusing on nutrient-dense foods and using healing recipes and meal plans that are tailored to their needs after surgery. For long-term health, experts may suggest eating a balanced diet, doing regular physical exercise, getting enough rest, and keeping up with medical follow-up to make sure a smooth recovery and the best health outcomes.

CHAPTER 3
SOUPS AND BREADS THAT HEAL

Soups and broths that help the body heal are very important for getting better after tubal ligation surgery. Even though this procedure is usually thought to be safe and not too invasive, it still needs some time to heal and recover. To repair tissues, get more energy, and stay healthy generally, the body needs to get enough food and water. Adding healthy soups and broths to your diet after surgery can help you get the nutrients, water, and support you need during this time.

Chicken Noodle Soup is a basic choice that not only tastes good but also is good for you in many ways. Usually, this soup has chicken, veggies, noodles, and a tasty broth. Protein, which is important for healing tissues and keeping your immune system strong, can be found in large amounts in chicken. Also, veggies like onions, carrots, and celery give you vitamins, minerals, and antioxidants that your body needs to heal and stay healthy. Not only does the soup add flavor, but it also helps you stay hydrated, which is very important for healing and avoiding problems. Adding whole-grain noodles to your diet adds complex carbohydrates that give you long-lasting energy to help you heal.

Another great choice for people who are healing from tubal ligation surgery is Soothing Bone Broth Recipes. When you boil animal bones and connective tissue for a long time, you get bone broth, which is a nutrient-rich liquid. There are minerals like calcium, magnesium, and phosphorus in this soup, as well as amino acids, collagen, and gelatin. All of these help the body heal and keep the gut healthy. Collagen and gelatin, which are found in bone broth, help organs heal, even ones that have been damaged by surgery. Regularly drinking bone broth can help lower inflammation, boost the immune system, and keep the gut system healthy, all of which are important for a full recovery.

The vegetable medley broth is full of nutrients that can help your diet after surgery and speed up the healing process. Carrots, celery, onions, garlic, and leafy greens are just some of the veggies that are simmered in water or low-sodium vegetable broth to make this broth. Including a variety of veggies in your diet will help you get a lot of different vitamins, minerals, antioxidants, and phytonutrients, all of which are important for helping the body heal. Also, veggies like carrots and leafy greens have a lot of vitamin C and beta-carotene, which are known to help the immune system. During the recovery time, drinking vegetable medley broth regularly can help restore lost nutrients, keep you hydrated, and improve your overall health.

soups and broths that help the body heal are great to add to a diet after tubal ligation. Chicken Noodle Soup is a comfort food that gives you protein, veggies, and carbs to help your body heal and give you energy. Collagen, amino acids, and minerals in Soothing Bone Broth Recipes help fix tissues, lower inflammation, and keep your gut healthy. Vegetable medley broth is a healthy choice that is full of the vitamins, minerals, and enzymes that your body needs to heal properly. Adding these healing soups and broths to your diet can help you get better faster and keep you healthy in the long run.

CHAPTER 4
BREAKFASTS THAT GIVE YOU ENERGY

Especially during the recovery time after tubal ligation surgery, breakfasts that give you energy are very important for getting your day going.

These meals should be made to give you long-lasting energy, and important nutrients, and help your body heal and stay healthy. Following a complete guide to the best post-surgery diet, like the Tubal Ligation Recovery Cookbook, makes sure that people get the nutrition they need to help them recover.

Breakfast bowls full of protein

People who have had tubal ligation surgery should eat breakfast bowls that are high in protein.

Protein is an important part of the diet after surgery because it helps repair tissues and build muscles.

You can make these food bowls your own by adding things like eggs, lean meats, tofu, beans, and nuts. This way, you can make sure you get enough protein. Whole grains like quinoa or brown rice add complex carbs that give you the energy that lasts, and veggies give you the vitamins, minerals, and fiber that your body needs. With avocado or olive oil drizzled on top, these breakfast bowls are not only healthy but also tasty and filling, making them a great choice for people who need a healthy start to the day.

Recipes for nutrient-dense smoothies

Another great choice for people who are recovering from tubal ligation surgery is smoothie recipes that are high in nutrients. Smoothies are great for people who have lost their appetite or are having digestive problems after surgery because they are easy to swallow. By mixing different fruits, leafy greens, and protein-rich foods like Greek yogurt or protein powder, people can make tasty and healthy smoothies that are full of vitamins, minerals, and antioxidants.

Adding healthy fats from avocado, nuts, or seeds makes the smoothie even healthier and more nutritious. It also makes you feel full and improves your health over time. These smoothies are full of healthy nutrients and can be eaten on their own for breakfast or with a small piece of whole-grain toast for a full and balanced meal.

Different kinds of healing porridge

Healing varieties of porridge are a comforting and healthy breakfast choice for people who have had tubal ligation surgery and are still healing.

Grains like oats, quinoa, and millet are used to make porridge. It is easy to stomach and can be changed by adding different things to make it healthier. Adding things like nuts, seeds, and dried fruits to the oats makes them healthier and gives it more protein, healthy fats, vitamins, and minerals. People can also add spices like ginger or cinnamon, which can help the body heal because they reduce inflammation. People can make healing porridge varieties that help them get better quickly and stay healthy for a long time by choosing whole grain choices and staying away from too much sugar or processed ingredients. Making and eating a warm bowl of nutritious porridge in the morning is a great way to start the day and helps the body heal after surgery.

CHAPTER 5
DRINKS AND TEA THAT ARE GOOD FOR YOU

Healing drinks and teas are very important for getting better after having tubal ligation surgery. During this time, the body goes through a lot of physical changes.

Drinking the right drinks can help ease pain, reduce inflammation, keep you hydrated, and boost your immune system. In this part, we'll talk about some healing drinks and teas that can help you recover faster after surgery.

Anti-inflammatory turmeric Tea is a strong drink that is famous for its amazing ability to reduce inflammation. Curcumin, a bioactive molecule found in turmeric, is known for its healing properties. Curcumin has strong anti-inflammatory and antioxidant qualities that can help reduce pain and swelling after surgery. Just put turmeric powder or newly grated turmeric root into hot water and let it steep for a while.

Add a bit of black pepper and a dash of honey or lemon to make it taste better and make it healthier. Regularly drinking turmeric tea can help reduce swelling, ease pain, and speed up the healing process generally.

Herbal infusions that hydrate are important for staying properly hydrated, especially during the healing phase. Dehydration can make your surgery effects worse and slow down your recovery.

Infusing herbs in water is a healthy way to stay hydrated that is also refreshing and nourishing. Herbs like chamomile, peppermint, and ginger can be soaked in hot water to make infusions that are soothing and good for you.

These herbal mixes not only help the body replace lost fluids, but they also help digestion, ease stomach pain, and encourage relaxation, all of which are important for healing.

Citrus drinks that boost your immune system are a great addition to your diet after surgery. The body's immune system may be briefly weakened after tubal ligation surgery, making it more likely to get infections and other illnesses.

Citrus fruits like oranges, lemons, and grapefruits have a lot of vitamin C, which is a powerful antioxidant that is known to help the immune system. Adding orange drinks to your diet can help boost your immune system and speed up the healing process. For a concentrated amount of vitamin C, freshly squeezed citrus juices, homemade lemonade, or water with citrus added to it are all great choices. In addition, these drinks keep you hydrated and cool while giving you a spicy, energizing taste.

Healing Drinks and Teas are important parts of the food for recovering from tubal ligation surgery.

Turmeric tea that reduces inflammation, herbal infusions that hydrate, and citrus drinks that boost immunity are all good for you in different ways. They can help with inflammation, hydration, and immunity. People who are getting tubal ligation surgery can help their bodies heal and stay healthy in the long run by adding these healing drinks to their daily meal plans.

CHAPTER 6
LUNCHES THAT HEAL

Following surgery for tubal ligation, it is very important to pay close attention to post-operative care, which includes food and nutrients.

A well-planned diet can make the mending process go much more smoothly, ensuring the best possible outcome and long-term health. This detailed guide to the best diet after surgery will talk about how important it is to eat healthy lunches and give you ideas for tasty quinoa salads, filling lentil soups, and fresh salad options that will help you feel better.

Restorative dinners are an important part of the recovery process after a tubal ligation because they provide the nutrients that help the body heal and give people their energy back. Care should be taken to make sure that these meals have the right amount of protein, fiber, vitamins, and minerals to help repair tissues, reduce inflammation, and improve general health.

Because they are versatile and full of nutrients, wholesome quinoa salads are a great choice for lunch after surgery. Quinoa is a gluten-free whole grain that is high in iron, magnesium, folate, protein, and fiber. It is also high in many vitamins and minerals. Adding quinoa to soups makes them filling and healthy, which helps the body recover. Quinoa is also a complete protein source because it has all nine necessary amino acids.

This makes it especially good for people who are trying to heal and rebuild their nutritional stores after surgery.

For lunch after a tubal ligation, satisfying lentil soup is a warm and healthy option. You can get a lot of protein, fiber, and important nutrients like calcium, iron, and potassium from lentils. Soups made with lentils can help keep blood sugar levels steady, make you feel full, and protect your gut health. Additionally, lentils contain phytonutrients that have anti-inflammatory qualities that can help ease pain after surgery and speed up the healing process.

Fresh salad combinations with a variety of colorful veggies, leafy greens, and healthy toppings are a great way to stay hydrated and refreshed after surgery.

Adding different colored veggies to salads makes sure that you get a wide range of vitamins, minerals, and antioxidants, which are important for keeping your immune system healthy and reducing inflammation. Adding lean protein sources like grilled chicken, tofu, or hard-boiled eggs to salads makes them healthier and more filling, which helps the body recover and stay healthy over time.

In conclusion, restorative lunches are an important part of the recovery process after a tubal ligation because they provide nutrition, support, and healing effects. Healthy quinoa salads, filling lentil soups, and fresh salad mixes are all great ways to make sure you get enough nutrients and stay healthy while you're recovering. By including these healthy meal choices in their diets after surgery, people can speed up the healing process, get more energy, and set themselves up for long-term health and vitality.

CHAPTER 7
FEEDING DINNER GUESTS

Dinners that are high in nutrients are very important for healing after tubal ligation surgery.

A healthy, well-balanced diet is important for healing, replacing nutrients lost, and maintaining general health. In this part, we'll talk about different dinner ideas that are meant to help with healing by providing comfort, nourishment, and support.

One-Pot Comfort Foods:

People who have had tubal ligation surgery often look for meals that are simple to make, comfortable to eat and don't require a lot of cleaning up.

One-pot meals are great because they are easy to make and don't skimp on taste or nutrition. For these meals, most of the time, all the ingredients are put together in one pot or pan.

This lets the flavors blend beautifully and reduces the amount of work needed for cooking and cleaning up.

Hearty soups, stews, and casseroles are all examples of comforting one-pot meals that can help you heal from surgery. You can make these dishes your own by adding different healthy foods like lean proteins, whole grains, and lots of veggies. Adding herbs and spices not only makes the food taste better, but they are also good for you because they fight inflammation and free radicals.

Fish and vegetable dishes that are high in nutrients: Adding fish and veggies to dinner recipes is a great way to get more nutrients and help your body heal and recover. Omega-3 fatty acids are found in large amounts in fish like salmon, trout, and mackerel. These acids help lower inflammation and keep your heart healthy. Fish is also a good source of protein, which is needed to repair tissues and keep the defence system working well.

When you eat fish with different coloured veggies, the meal is even healthier because the vegetables provide more vitamins, minerals, and antioxidants. When you roast or grill fish and veggies together, it's easy to prepare and clean up, and the flavors and textures stay the same. Adding herbs, citrus zest, and healthy fats like olive oil to these meals makes them taste better without taking away from their health benefits.

Easy dinner ideas with plant-based protein:

For people who are on a plant-based diet or want to eat more plant-based meals, many choices can help them recover from surgery. Beans, lentils, tofu, tempeh, and edamame are all plant-based proteins that are high in fiber, vitamins, minerals, and phytonutrients. This makes them great choices for supporting healing and general health.

Hearty salads, stir-fries, grain bowls, and vegetable-based stews are all plant-based protein dinner ideas.

These foods have a lot of different tastes and textures, and they are also full of nutrients that help the body heal. Including a range of plant-based proteins also makes sure that people get all the important amino acids they need for good health and recovery.

healthy foods are very important for getting better after tubal ligation surgery. Comforting one-pot meals, fish and veggie dishes that are high in nutrients, and plant-based protein dinner ideas are all tasty and healthy ways to help with healing and long-term health. People can make their post-surgery diets better for recovery and general health by focusing on nutrient-dense foods and tasty combinations.

CHAPTER 8
SNACKS AND TREATS THAT HEAL

Snacks and treats that help you heal are very important for getting better after tubal ligation surgery. Not only are these snacks tasty, but they are also full of nutrients that help the body heal and stay healthy. It's important to know how to nourish the body during this time of healing if you want to get better quickly and easily. With a focus on giving the best nutrition, the snacks and treats below have been carefully chosen to help with healing and promote long-term health.

The nut butter energy balls are:

Nut butter energy balls are a healthy and easy-to-carry snack for people who have had tubal ligation surgery. Nut butter, rolled oats, seeds, and sweetness like honey or maple syrup are often mixed to make these little treats.

Almond, peanut, and cashew butter are good sources of protein and healthy fats that your body needs to fix tissues and keep your immune system strong. Rolled oats add fiber, which helps your body digest food and gives you energy all day.

Also, omega-3 fatty acids and minerals found in seeds like flaxseed and chia are good for the body's healing processes. By including nut butter energy balls in a person's diet after surgery, they can enjoy a snack that makes them feel full and gives them the nutrients they need to heal.

Sticks of crisp vegetables with hummus:

Crispy vegetable sticks with hummus make a healthy and refreshing snack for people who have had tubal ligation surgery and are still healing.

The crunchiness of fresh vegetables and the softness of hummus come together in this snack to make a tasty and healthy treat. There are a lot of vitamins, minerals, and antioxidants in vegetables like celery, bell peppers, carrots, and onions.

These are very important for keeping the immune system strong and lowering inflammation.

Using beans, tahini, olive oil, and lemon juice to make hummus gives you protein, fiber, and healthy fats that help you feel full and keep your digestive system healthy. Mixed together, crunchy vegetable sticks and hummus make a healthy snack that helps the body heal better after surgery.

Dark chocolate treats that are good for you:

Dark chocolate treats with antioxidants are a tasty and healthy treat for people who have had tubal ligation surgery. Because it has a lot of cocoa, dark chocolate is full of antioxidants like flavonoids and polyphenols.

These have been linked to many health benefits, such as better heart health and less inflammation. When you choose dark chocolate with a high cocoa percentage, you get the most antioxidants and the least amount of extra sugar. Dark chocolate also has minerals in it, such as iron, magnesium, and zinc, which are needed to make energy, keep muscles working, and protect the immune system. Including dark chocolate antioxidant treats in your diet after surgery is a tasty way to fill your cravings while also improving your health and helping your body heal.

 healing snacks and treats are very important for getting better after tubal ligation surgery.

Nut butter energy balls, crisp veggie sticks with hummus, and dark chocolate antioxidant treats are all tasty and healthy ways to help your body heal and stay healthy over time. By adding these snacks to their diet after surgery, people can give their bodies the nutrients they need to heal and improve their general health while they are recovering.

CHAPTER 9
HERBAL REMEDIES FOR HEALING

As interest in natural healing methods and holistic health practices grows, the idea of using herbal remedies to help people recover from surgery has gained steam. This is especially true after a tubal ligation. You can help your body heal naturally with herbal treatments that are gentle but effective.

They can ease pain, help digestion, boost the immune system, and promote relaxation.

Using herbal remedies as part of a recovery plan can improve general health and make the healing process go more smoothly.

Tea with Lavender to Relax

People love lavender tea, which comes from the sweet lavender plant. It is known for helping people relax and calm down. Patients who have had tubal ligation surgery may feel more stressed or anxious afterward, which can slow down the mending process. Having lavender tea can help ease these feelings and make you feel cool and peaceful. Essential oils like lavender contain chemicals like linalool and linalyl acetate that have been shown to help calm people down and make them feel less anxious. Patients can successfully control their stress levels and speed up the healing process by adding soothing lavender tea to their post-surgery recovery routine.

Herbal infusions for digestion

After treatment, like tubal ligation, many people have digestive problems like bloating, gas, and constipation. Herbal drinks made with digestive herbs can help ease these symptoms and keep your digestive system healthy while you're healing. Carminative ingredients include peppermint, ginger, fennel, and chamomile. This means that they can help get rid of gas and bloating while also soothing the digestive system. Peppermint, in particular, has menthol in it, which relaxes the muscles in the digestive system.

This makes digestion easier and less painful.

By adding digestive plant infusions to their diet, patients can ease digestive pain and keep their digestive system working at its best while they are healing.

Herbal blends that boost the immune system

To avoid getting infections and speed up the healing process after tubal ligation surgery, it is important to support the immune system.

Herbal blends that boost the immune system and are full of antioxidants, vitamins, and minerals can help the body's natural defences work better and improve general health. Ingredients like echinacea, berries, astragalus, and ginger are known for their immune-boosting effects and ability to make the immune system work better. For example, echinacea has chemicals in it that make immune cells work harder, which helps the body fight off diseases better.

Flavonoids and other antioxidants found in large amounts in elderberry can help reduce swelling and boost the immune system. Patients getting tubal ligation surgery can boost their immune systems and speed up the healing process by adding immune-boosting herbal mixes to their diet.

herbal remedies can be a useful addition to standard medical treatments for helping people recover from surgery, such as tubal ligation. Relaxing lavender tea can help you deal with worry and calm down, and digestive herbal infusions can ease stomach pain and improve digestive health. Herbal mixes that boost the immune system can help the body's natural defences work better and speed up the healing process. Patients can speed up their recovery and improve their health in the long run by using these herbal remedies as part of their recovery plan.

CHAPTER 10
MINDFUL EATING AND TAKING CARE OF YOURSELF

Being mindful about what you eat and taking care of yourself is very important during the recovery process after surgery, especially after a treatment like tubal ligation. Being fully present and aware of the food you eat, the feelings you have while eating, and the cues your body sends about hunger and fullness are all parts of mindful eating. It's not just about what you eat; it's also about how you eat and how you feel about food. In the same way, self-care means taking care of your physical, emotional, and mental health to help you heal and stay healthy generally.

Why mindful eating is important

Eating mindfully is a very important part of getting better after tubal ligation surgery. After this kind of surgery, the body needs the best nutrition to help it heal and get stronger.

Mindful eating tells people to take their time and enjoy every bite, which helps their bodies handle food better and absorb nutrients. It helps you keep a healthy weight, which is important for your health in general and especially after surgery.

Mindful eating keeps you from overeating or undereating by letting you know when you're full. This makes sure that your body gets enough food for the healing phase. Mindful eating also helps you have a good relationship with food, which makes it less likely that you'll use food as a way to deal with stress or mental problems that are common during recovery.

Techniques for Recovering from Stress

Many physical and mental things can make recovery from tubal ligation surgery more difficult.

Not only does stress slow down the mending process, but it can also make pain worse and cause you to take longer to recover.

So, it's important to include techniques for relieving stress in your daily life. Deep breathing, meditation, and easy yoga are all activities that can help you relax and deal with stress. Deep breathing routines, for example, make the body's relaxation response work, which lowers blood pressure and heart rate. Meditation can help calm the mind and make it easier to think clearly. Gentle yoga moves can help the body release tension and improve circulation. These methods not only lessen the physical effects of stress, but they also make people stronger emotionally, which helps them deal with the challenges of recovery better.

Methods of Self-Care for Healing

Self-care routines include many different things that people do to improve their physical, emotional, and mental health. Self-care is very important for healing and getting back to a healthy balance after a tubal closure.

Physical self-care means taking care of your body's needs, like making sure you get enough rest, stay hydrated, and do gentle moving or exercise as your doctor tells you to. Emotional self-care means recognizing and dealing with any feelings that come up during healing, whether they are anxious, angry, or sad.

 This can be done by writing in a diary, getting help from friends or family or a therapist, and being kind to yourself. Psychological self-care means taking care of your mental health by doing things that make you happy and satisfied, like hobbies, artistic activities, or spending time in nature.

People who are recovering from tubal ligation can build resilience, boost their immune system, and speed up the healing process by putting themselves first.

This will eventually lead to long-term health.

CHAPTER 11
BUILDING HEALTHY HABITS AFTER RECOVERY

In addition to rest and medical care, people who have had tubal ligation surgery need to pay attention to their nutrition to help them heal and stay healthy in the long run. The path to a full recovery doesn't end when you leave the hospital or finish your post-surgery care. For long-term health, it's important to know how to keep good habits after recovery. In this detailed guide, we'll talk about how important it is to switch to healthy eating habits that will last, keep your nutrient balance after healing, and make exercise and movement a regular part of your life.

Changing to healthy eating habits that will last

Getting back to long-term healthy eating habits after tubal ligation surgery is very important for your health and well-being as a whole.

You need to make sure your body gets enough nutrients while you're healing so it can get stronger again. But it's just as important to keep eating nutrient-dense foods even after you're better to stay healthy in the long term. To make this change, you need to eat a balanced diet with lots of different fruits, veggies, whole grains, lean proteins, and healthy fats.

Adding a variety of nutrient-rich foods to your daily meals is one of the most important things you can do to start eating healthier in the long run. Include a lot of different coloured fruits and veggies in your diet. They are full of vitamins, minerals, and antioxidants that are good for your health and immune system. Whole grains like oats, quinoa, and brown rice give you long-lasting energy and fiber, which helps your body digest food and keep a healthy weight.

Along with eating more whole foods, it's important to watch your portion amounts and not eat too many processed foods, sugary snacks, or fats that are bad for you.

Choose lean proteins like chicken, fish, tofu, and beans to help your muscles heal and keep you full. Getting healthy fats from foods like olive oil, nuts, seeds, avocados, and avocados can help lower inflammation and keep your heart healthy.

Planning meals ahead of time is very important for making the change to healthy eating habits that will last, especially during the healing period when energy levels may be lower. You can make sure you have access to healthy foods even on busy days by planning and making healthy meals ahead of time. Try out new flavors and recipes to keep your meals interesting and fun. This will help you stick to your long-term diet goals.

Keeping the balance of nutrients after healing is important for keeping your health in general and avoiding nutritional deficiencies.

After tubal ligation surgery, your body may temporarily not be able to receive certain nutrients, or it may need extra nutrients to help it heal. Because of this, it's important to watch what you eat and make sure you're meeting your body's food needs every day.

Protein is one of the most important nutrients to pay attention to after healing because it helps repair tissues and muscles. Eating enough protein-rich foods, like lean meats, chicken, fish, eggs, dairy, tofu, and legumes, can help your body heal and keep you from losing muscle. To get the most out of protein, try to spread it out evenly throughout the day.

To improve your health and immunity, it's important to eat a range of vitamins and minerals as well as protein.

Vitamin C is needed to make collagen and help wounds heal. You can find it in citrus foods, strawberries, bell peppers, and broccoli. Vitamin D helps keep bones healthy and the immune system working well.

You can get it from the sun and foods that have been treated with it. To keep your bones and teeth strong, you need to eat calcium-rich foods like cheese, leafy greens, and plant-based foods that have been fortified.

Flaxseeds, chia seeds, peanuts, and fatty fish are all good sources of omega-3 fatty acids. They can help lower inflammation and keep your heart healthy. Iron-rich foods like lean red meat, poultry, fish, lentils, beans, and cereals with added iron are important for avoiding iron deficiency anemia, especially in women who are having their periods.

Eating a mix of fruits, vegetables, whole grains, and healthy fats can help you get all the nutrients you need for good health and well-being.

To improve your physical and mental health after tubal ligation surgery, you need to make exercise and moving a part of your daily life.

During the recovery time, it's important to listen to your body and get enough rest. However, slowly getting back into physical activity can help improve your strength, flexibility, and overall fitness level.

Low-impact activities like walking, swimming, yoga, and cycling are great for recovering from surgery because they are easy on the body and can be changed to fit your fitness level and comfort. Start with short, easy workouts and slowly add more time and effort as you get stronger and more confident. To avoid getting hurt and speed up the healing process, remember to warm up properly before working out and cool down properly afterward.

Using light weights, resistance bands, or your body weight for strength training can help you build muscle and change the way your body looks generally. To improve your steadiness and ability to move around normally, work on big muscle groups like your legs, arms, back, and core. Flexibility workouts like yoga, Pilates, and stretching can help improve your range of motion, ease muscle tension, and make you more flexible overall.

Pay attention to your body and any signs of pain or soreness while you work out. If you feel any pain or soreness, stop doing what you're doing right away and talk to your doctor before starting again. During the early stages of healing, it's important to take things slowly and not push yourself too hard.

Find ways to move throughout your daily life in addition to scheduled exercise sessions to boost your general activity levels and support a healthy lifestyle. During breaks at work, go for short walks or take the stairs instead of the lift. You can also do fun things like dancing, gardening, or sports with family and friends.

Not only is regular exercise good for your body, but it's also a key part of dealing with stress, lifting your mood, and making your life better in general.

Try to do a lot of different things that you enjoy and that fit with your fitness goals and hobbies. After tubal ligation surgery, you can help your long-term healing and keep your health and well-being at their best by making regular exercise and movement a priority.

CONCLUSION

Recovery from surgery, especially tubal ligation, is more than just getting better physically. It's also about taking care of your mind and body for long-term health. This whole guide has talked a lot about how important eating is during recovery and given you a lot of tools, like healing recipes and expert advice, to help you.

In each chapter, we've talked about how important it is to get enough water, protein-rich foods, healthy fats, and key nutrients for healing.

Each recipe and idea has been carefully chosen to help you heal and give your body the food and nutrients it needs. There are comforting soups and broths, energizing breakfasts, healing drinks, healthy lunches, and dinners, as well as healthy snacks and treats.

To help with a complete recovery, we've also talked about the benefits of herbal remedies, mindful eating, and self-care methods. Since we know that recovery doesn't end right after surgery, we've also talked about how important it is to build healthy habits for long-term health.

For example, switching to a balanced diet, making sure you get enough nutrients, and making regular exercise and movement a part of your daily life.

As you start to heal, remember that taking care of yourself and eating well is not only important for rehab but also for living a healthy, happy life.

Take the advice in this complete guide to heart, and may you find strength, perseverance, and a new life as you move through this part of your life and beyond.